Natural Cures

Herbal Medicine for Natural Remedies at Home

Gaia Rodale

Just to say Thank You for Purchasing this Book I want to give you a gift <u>100% absolutely FREE</u>

A Copy of My Upcoming Special Report *"The Organic Gardener's Calendar: Monthly 'To Dos' for Beginner Gardeners"*

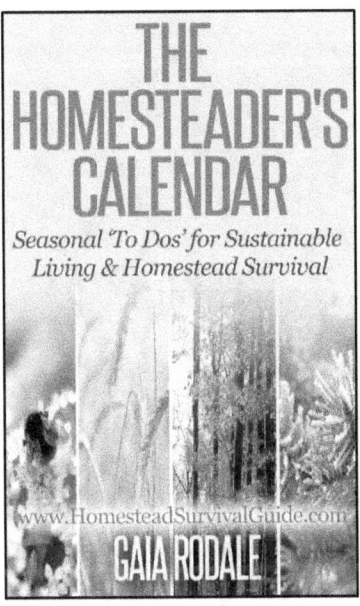

Go to <u>www.HomesteadSurvivalGuide.com</u> to Reserve Your FREE Copy Today

Table of Contents

Introduction

I want to thank you and congratulate you for purchasing, *"Natural Cures, Herbal Medicine for Natural Remedies at Home."*

For thousands of years, women have stocked their stillrooms with herbs, spices, tinctures, infusions, oils, and ointments in order to treat the various illnesses and ailments of their family.

With the rapid advances in modern medicine over the past century, most of this knowledge and experience has fallen by the wayside. However, there is still benefit to be had in learning to grow, make, and use your own herbal remedies.

For many families, making herbal remedies just makes good sense. Most of the ingredients can easily be produced in a small herb garden, which can lead to a real cost reduction over time.

While we have the benefit of modern medicine treat the emergencies, that doesn't mean we have to be completely reliant on that single solution.

Making your own herbal remedies isn't difficult, you just need a basic understanding of the types of remedies most commonly used, how to make them, and which herbs are beneficial for treating which problems.

This guide provides you with all that information, which means you will be ready to start infusing and decocting soon!

From explaining the different types of remedies to providing some easy beginner recipes for making remedies to treat various ailments, this guide gives you the foundational understanding and beginner basics to get your herbal remedy efforts off the ground.

Happy Homesteading!

Gaia Rodale

Why Choose the Natural Path

One of the most important things we have lost in modern society, at least in my opinion, is the stillroom. This room, which was dedicated to holding the herbs, salves, recipes, tinctures, and other ingredients used to treat everyday ailments, used to be found in every rural homestead. In fact, if you went back in time, you would find stillrooms in every kind of dwelling from the castles of medieval times to the abbeys of the ancient church.

Our move away from herbal medicine and fostering the knowledge to treat illness and disease naturally has only come in the last 150 years as modern medical practices have rapidly advanced. Don't get me wrong, I am not decrying the amazing abilities of modern medicine to do things that our ancestors would never have thought possible. There is a reason we no longer call strep throat morbid sore throat; namely, people are no longer at great risk of dying from it. However, as the wonders of modern medicine have swept across the Western world, our society has lost touch with and lost faith in the remedies and treatments that people used to attend to their health for thousands of years.

While there are definitely some areas where modern medicine will always be better, more and more herbal or natural options are being shown to be just as effective as the pharmaceuticals espoused by modern medicine. This means that in many cases, we have the means to mend ourselves without having to visit a doctor or ingest a bunch of chemicals. With a little knowledge and some extra effort, we can make herbal remedies to deal with some of our basic health problems.

Why Herbal Medicine is a Good Fit for Your Family

Herbal remedies and natural medicine are a natural fit for
those working to build a sustainable, self-sufficient lifestyle.
Most homesteaders have gardens. By simply adding a few
herbs here and there you can grow your own basic pharmacy!

Learning to use herbal medicine to treat basic health
problems like colds, stomach problems, and aches and pains
increases your self-sufficiency. Knowing that you can whip
up a batch of ginger tea to treat a tummy ache makes you
more independent. Knowing when you can treat things
yourself and when it is time to see a doctor actually helps
decrease your dependence on modern medicine.

When you can use an herb that you grew yourself to make a
tea or a poultice or a ointment to treat yourself, you are
saving money. You are saving the cost of buying
pharmaceutical treatments at the store and the cost of any co-
pay or fee to see a doctor.

Practicing natural medicine and using herbal remedies also
makes you more aligned with nature and the world around
you. You know every ingredient that goes into each remedy
you make. Also, there is a good chance that you made or
grew the ingredients as well which means you know their
origins.

Benefits of Herbal Remedies

One of the biggest advantages of using herbal remedies is
that you can grow the ingredients you need to make them in
your own garden. This cuts down on costs. It also gives you
full control and knowledge of what you are putting in your
body and those of your loved ones.

Natural Cures

Many of the pharmaceuticals used to treat basic ailments were derived from the same herbs used in the herbal remedies that are most effective in treating those ailments. This means that despite the fact that there isn't enough research to support the efficacy of many herbal remedies, they are clearly effective because the medicine that comes in a bottle from the drug store has the herbal remedy as its ancestor. For example, aspirin was originally derived from the bark of willow trees, the same bark used by herbalists to treat headache.

Another important benefit of choosing herbal remedies when appropriate is that they generally have fewer side effects than their pharmaceutical counterparts. Natural medicine and herbal remedies can also do a better job of treating chronic conditions that don't respond well to modern medical treatments.

Finally, herbal remedies are simply more available. While I cannot manufacture Pepto-Bismol in my kitchen, I can make a ginger infusion. The ingredients for herbal remedies are easy to find and easy to grow, and the remedies themselves are often simplistic to create. This makes them ideal for those in rural areas or for families who are looking to rely less on the modern healthcare system

However, I do want to stress that while I think every family should embrace herbal remedies that can be used to treat common ailments, I am not saying they are a replacement for regular medical care or modern medical treatments; at least, not all of them.

As I said before, there will always be medical problems that modern medicine is more able to deal with. Emergency situations, life-threatening diseases, and chronic debilitating conditions are all examples of where modern medicine must play a role.

However, I strongly believe that there is a place for herbal medicine in that picture as well. The key is finding the right balance and using herbal remedies and natural medicine where it makes sense.

Growing Your Own Herbs

If you have had the chance to read any of my books in the *Organic Gardening Beginners Planting Guide* series, you know that I am an avid gardener, and that I grow a lot of herbs myself. If you haven't had a chance to check this series out, I recommend grabbing *Organic Herb Gardening: the Beginners Guide to Planning, Growing, and Preserving Your Own Culinary and Medicinal Herbs* first as it provides a wealth of information on how to grow your own herbs organically.

Some of the reasons I think every homesteader and gardener should grow their own organic herbs are:

- When you grow your own herbs you know how they were grown and what was used to grow them. This is imperative when you are putting something in your body.
- Knowing that the herbs you grow are free of harmful chemical residue can give you piece of mind when using them to create herbal remedies.
- When you use organic herbs for culinary or medicinal purposes, you decrease your lifetime exposure to synthetic chemicals.
- Organic herb gardening practices also focus on resource conservation which means being conscious of the use of resources like water.
- Growing your own herbs saves money, especially if you learn to save the seeds for use in future years.

Growing a Medicinal Herb Garden

You can easily include herbs in your garden. Further, simply growing them can offer additional benefits to the rest of your garden. Many herbs are excellent companions for vegetables because they offer natural pest control benefits and help boost everything from flavor to yield.

You can also create a special herb garden geared towards growing plants for medicinal purposes. One of my favorite ways to do this is included in the organic herb garden guide mentioned above. It is called a Medicine Wheel garden, and it is laid out in a circle with eight segments. Each segment holds the plants used to treat a specific type of medical problem. This makes it easy to know your go-to herbs for different medical purposes.

Some examples of the sections from a Medicine Wheel garden and the herbs that are grown in that section are:

- Nervous – Remedies for the nervous system feature chamomile, lemon balm, and valerian
- Respiratory – Remedies to treat the respiratory system feature mint, sage, and thyme
- Digestive – Remedies to treat the digestive system feature dill, peppermint, and dandelion

For more details about what is included in a Medicine Wheel Herb garden and how to build one, read my *Organic Herb Gardening* book.

Making Your Own Herbal Remedies

Whether you choose to grow your own herbs or purchase them from a high quality supply, you will need to know the basic ways that herbs are used medicinally. Each of the common types of herbal remedies and instructions on how to make them are outlined below.

Essential Oils

Essential oils, which are the extracted oils of plant material, are a common form of herbal remedy. There are three ways to create the substance most people refer to as essential oil, although only the distillation method, which is not recommended for home use, produces true essential oils.

Distillation

Distillation can be done one of three ways. It can be done with the plant material being boiled in water, the steam collected, and the oils extracted from the water. It can be done with water and steam, where boiling water and steam are forced through a container filled with plant matter. The steam is then collected, and the oils are separated from the water. It can also be done with just steam, where the steam is forced through the container of plant material, collected, and the oils are separated from the water.

To make essential oils with steam distillation, you will need a still like this one that can be purchased online: 2000ml Steam Distillation Essential Oil Extractor. Then follow these instructions.

1. Set up the still.
2. Fill the boiling water container with water.
3. Add boiling stones to the water.

4. Add dried plant matter to the plant matter container. Pack it tightly, but not so tightly that the steam won't be able to pass through it.
5. Start cool water flow into the condenser.
6. Turn on the heat source that will boil the water in the boiling container.
7. Monitor the water level in the boiling container to ensure it remains 1/3-2/3 full throughout the process.
8. Continue boiling until plant matter has shrinks considerably, usually 30-45 minutes.
9. Carefully separate the water from the essential oil by pouring the water out from under the oil.
10. Move the oil to a dark-colored glass bottle.

Cold Pressing

This method is primarily used for extracting oils from citrus rinds and results in expressed oil which is not exactly the same as an essential oil.

To obtain expressed oils by cold pressing:

1. Remove the peels from the fruit, wash them, dry them, and place them on a cookie sheet.
2. Heat oven to 120°F, and heat the peels for 2 hours.
3. Remove the rinds, and use a garlic press to press the oil out of the rind into a container.

Extraction

This method is used to create absolutes which are similar to, but not the same as essential oils. Extraction requires the use of a solvent. In the instructions below, high proof alcohol is used as the solvent.

1. Put plant material in a canning jar, and pour grain alcohol of 120-190 proof over the materials until they are just covered.
2. Put the lid on the jar and shake vigorously for several minutes.
3. Place the jar somewhere out of the sun to steep.
4. Continue shaking the jar for several minutes three times a day until the plant material starts to lose its color. This generally takes 2-6 days.
5. Strain the liquid with a strainer to remove the plant material.
6. Put the strained plant material in some cheesecloth and squeeze any remaining liquid out to capture all the liquid.
7. Put all the liquid back in a clean canning jar, put the lid on, and let it sit for a couple days until it starts to separate.
8. Once you see the oil separate from the alcohol, place the jar in the freezer.
9. When the oil and any plant gunk have frozen solid (the alcohol won't freeze), remove the jar from the freezer, and separate the solid oils from the gunk and the unfrozen alcohol.
10. Return the jar to the freezer, and repeat the preceding step.

11. Store the extracted oil in a dark-colored glass bottle.

You can also distill the steeped alcohol/oil mixture to extract the oils.

Lotions and Creams

Lotions and creams are used to create herbal remedies that are absorbed into the skin. They generally consist of some type of oil and water. They can be made with or without emulsifiers which are agents that help liquids or other substances that don't mix well remain stable in their mixed state. Some of the most common emulsifiers are:

- Beeswax which helps thicken lotions and creams
- Lecithin which makes lotions and creams more slippery
- Lanolin which helps thicken lotions and creams
- Glycerin which helps make creams and lotions more moisturizing

To make a basic lotion:

1. Heat ¾ cup of coconut oil and ½ ounce of beeswax until melted, then cool until it looks filmy.
2. Pour 1 cup of water into the blender.
3. Turn blender on low, and add the melted mixture slowly to the water.
4. Once all the melted mixture has been added to the water, put the cover on the blender and turn up the speed.
5. Add any other ingredients at this point.
6. Blend until you have a creamy lotion texture.
7. Remove from the blender, and store in a jar in the fridge.

To make a basic cream, follow the same process as above, but use an ounce of beeswax and ¾ cup of water.

Infusions

An infusion is made by steeping plant matter in hot water. The most common and familiar type of infusion is tea. Infusions contain extracted vitamins and other substances that can be beneficial as herbal remedies.

Infusions are simple to make using the following instructions:

1. Measure out the amount of water you need based on the amount of herbs you are using. One tablespoon of herbs needs one cup of water.
2. Boil the water.
3. Pour the boiling water over the herbs, and let steep. The amount of steeping time will vary depending on how much infusion you are making. A good rule of thumb is 15-30 minutes per tablespoon of herbs.
4. Strain and reserve liquid.
5. Store in the refrigerator.

Decoctions

Decoctions are generally used to extract the medicinal substances from plants with heavy stems, roots, leaves, or bark. This method is generally used to make tinctures. The plant material is mashed or crushed and then boiled or simmered in liquid for a long period of time, which enables more of the plants oils to be released into the liquid.

To make a basic decoction:

1. Mash or crush the plant material to be used to better enable the medicinal properties to be released.
2. Add the plant material to a pot of water, and bring to a boil.
3. Boil for at least 10 minutes and for as long as one hour. Longer boiling times will create stronger decoctions.
4. Strain and reserve the liquid. Discard the plant material.

Poultices

A poultice is an external treatment, generally made from some kind of plant material, that is applied directly to the skin or to an injury to allow the medicinal properties of the herbs to be absorbed into the skin.

To make a basic poultice from dried herbs:

1. Grind the herbs down to a powder.
2. Place herbs in a bowl, and add enough warm water to make the ground herbs into a paste.
3. Clean the area of the body where the poultice will be applied.
4. You can either spread the poultice out directly on the skin or place a thin layer of clean fabric over the skin and then apply the poultice.
5. Cover the poultice with a thin cloth and then cover with plastic wrap and tape in place with medical tape.

Poultices can be kept in place for one hour up to 24 hours, as needed. You may need to apply fresh poultices several times to achieve the desired result.

Ointments

Ointments are used for many herbal remedies and are similar to lotions and creams. They are relatively easy to make.

How to make an herbal ointment:

1. Heat the oven to 200°F.
2. Place one cup of the oil of your choice and one cup of the herbs you are using in a double boiler, and heat over medium heat.
3. Once the oven is at 200°F, turn it off.
4. Heat the oil and herb mixture for several minutes until it is heated through. Do not let it boil.
5. Take the top half of the double boiler, and put it in the oven for three hours.
6. Remove the pan from the oven, and strain using cheese cloth.
7. Pour the oil back into the double boiler pan, and place both pieces back on the stove over medium heat.
8. Add ¼ cup of bees wax to the oil.
9. Stir until wax melts into the oil.
10. Pour into a glass jar, and allow to cool before putting on the lid.

Treating the Common Cold

The common cold comes with several tell-tale symptoms that all need to be treated in order to get some relief until the illness passes. These symptoms are:

- Runny or stuffy nose
- Sore throat
- Cough
- Congestion
- Low-grade fever

Slight body aches or mild headaches are also symptoms, but those will be covered in the next section. To help keep the cold from taking hold and to shorten its stay, take one tablespoon of virgin coconut oil every day as soon as symptoms appear.

Runny or Stuffy Nose

Peppermint Remedies

Peppermint is often used in commercial cold remedies because of its decongesting powers. You can create peppermint essential oil, place it on a cotton ball or dish towel, and breathe in the fumes. You can also create a peppermint-based salve to rub on the chest to aid with decongestion. A peppermint infusion for drinking is another way to use peppermint to help alleviate a stuffy nose.

Sage and Honey Solution

Another way to treat a runny nose is to add a pinch of dried, ground sage to a teaspoon of honey. No need for mixing or mashing. The sage will help dry up the sinuses.

Sore Throat

Marshmallow Root Infusion

One of the best ways to treat a sore throat is with an infusion of marshmallow root. Make a standard infusion using one tablespoon of dried marshmallow root to one cup of water. Steep the mixture for at least 30 minutes before straining. You can re-warm the liquid before drinking if desired.

Licorice Root Decoction

A licorice root decoction will also help soothe a sore throat. To make this remedy, you will need

- 1 cup chopped dry licorice root
- 1/2 cup cinnamon chips
- 2 tablespoons whole cloves
- 1/2 cup dried chamomile flowers

Combine all the ingredients in a bowl. Measure out about 3 tablespoons, and put in a pan. Add 2.5-3 cups of cool water to the pan. Heat to boiling, and then simmer for 10 minutes before straining and drinking.

Cough

Generally, when we treat a cough, we use cough syrup and cough drops. Here are recipes for making an herbal version of each.

Honey Sage Cough Syrup

- 1 cup honey
- 1 tablespoon fresh squeezed lemon juice
- 1 teaspoon dried sage
- 1 teaspoon dried horehound

To make this decoction, combine all ingredients in a pan and stir over medium heat until they simmer. Remove from heat and cover. Allow to sit and steep for 15 minutes. Strain liquid, discard solids, and bottle. Keep finished syrup in the refrigerator for up to 6 months. Give a tablespoon at a time as needed. Not suitable for children 2 and under.

Honey Horehound Cough Drops

- ¼ cup dried horehound
- 1 cup water
- 2 cups sugar
- 2 tablespoons honey

Add water and herbs to a saucepan and simmer, covered, for 20 minutes. Strain solids and discard. Return infused water to the pot. Add sugar and honey and bring to a boil, stirring frequently. Check the temp with a candy thermometer. Boil until the mixture reaches 330°F. Continue stirring throughout. As the mixture approaches this temperature, check to see if it is becoming thread. Pull the spoon out, and see if the mix forms a thread between the bottom of the spoon and the mixture in the pot. Once it threads, drop a couple drops into a cup of cold water. Take the drops out of the water and bite into one. If it is sticky, keep going. If it crackles, turn off the heat.

Once the cough drops reach this hard-crack stage, pour the mixture out onto a baking sheet lined with parchment paper. Let the mixture cool. Before the drops completely harden, score out the drops with a knife, so they will be easy to break them apart once they are completely hardened. Wrap individual drops in parchment paper or plastic wrap and store.

Congestion

Mustard Poultice

Mustard poultices can be beneficial in treating congestion, especially in the chest. This was one of the ways our forefathers treated the congestion seen with pneumonia. When using a mustard poultice, always place a cloth between the poultice and the skin because mustard can be a skin irritant.

To make a mustard poultice, grind up dried mustard seed into a powder. Combine 2 tablespoons of mustard powder and two tablespoons of baking soda in a small bowl. Add water to create a paste, and apply the poultice to the chest.

Eucalyptus Sage Infusion

Another great way to treat congestion is with an infusion of eucalyptus and sage. Make a standard infusion using 1 tablespoon of dried eucalyptus leaves, 1 tablespoon of dried sage, and 3 cups of water. Steep the mixture for at least 15-

30 minutes before straining. You can re-warm the liquid before drinking if desired.

Low Grade Fever

Yarrow Infusion

Yarrow can help break a fever by inducing sweating which helps bring the fever to an end. Make a standard infusion with 1 tablespoon of dried yarrow and 1 cup of boiling water. Steep for 10 minutes. It may take more than one cup of this infusion to get you sweating.

Garlic Poultice

A garlic poultice applied to the bottoms of the feet can help bring down a fever. Use fresh cloves of garlic that are mashed into a paste with olive oil to make the poultice. Do not apply directly to the skin as garlic can be an irritant. Use a thin clean cloth against the skin, apply the poultice over the cloth, and then wrap in gauze and leave overnight.

Herbs that Help Common Cold Symptoms

Astragalus Root

Astragalus is used as a preventative measure against viral infection and can be taken at the start of a cold or flu to help shorten the length of the ailment by bolstering the immune system.

Birch Bark & Leaf

Birch tree bark contains salicylate like white willow bark and was another precursor to modern day aspirin.

Echinacea

Echinacea is also used to boost the immune system and is often taken during cold and flu season to prevent these ailments.

Elderberry

Elderberries when decocted into syrup can be used to treat colds and diarrhea. In infusion form, they are believed to be beneficial in fighting viruses like the flu.

Eucalyptus

Eucalyptus is very beneficial when used in cold and congestion remedies. Eucalyptus oil can also be used as a pain reliever for sore muscles and arthritis pain.

Fennel Seed

Fennel seed can be used in remedies for treating coughs. It can also help with hormonal problems seen in menopause.

Thyme

Thyme is one of the best herbs to treat colds and coughs. It can address most cold symptoms and helps clear congestion from the lungs.

Dealing with Aches and Pains

Headaches, body aches, and even joint pain can be everyday occurrences or accompany other ailments as a symptom. Either way, you need to be able to alleviate them in order to feel better and get back to your day. These options will provide relief to different kinds of aches and pains.

Body Aches

Arnica Ointment

Arnica can be beneficial for soothing sore muscles. It is even helpful is easing the pain associated with sprains. It can also be used to speed up the healing of bruises. It should not be used on broken skin or be used to alleviate the pain associated with cuts or scrapes.

- 2 cups coconut oil
- 1 ounce dried arnica flowers
- ¾ cup beeswax

Follow the standard recipe for creating an ointment with the following exceptions:

- Before adding the flowers to the oil, chop, crush, or mash them up a little to help release the medicinal properties faster.
- You will want to steep the oil and herb mixture for 12-24 hours. You can do this by using the lowest setting on your oven to keep them heated while steeping or by using a Crockpot.

Lemongrass, Peppermint, and Marjoram Oil

This mixture of essential oils/absolutes can be beneficial in treating muscle cramps. Create the base essential oils or absolutes with the method of your choice. Then combine 3-5 drops of each with a tablespoon of olive oil to dilute. Rub the oil into the affected area.

Basil, Chamomile, and Marjoram Oil

This mixture of essential oils/absolutes can be beneficial in treating muscle spasms. Create the base essential oils or absolutes with the method of your choice. Then combine 3-5 drops of each with a tablespoon of olive oil to dilute. Rub the oil into the affected area.

Stinging Nettle Infusion

Stinging nettles can be beneficial for easing the pain associated with arthritis and gout. Make a standard infusion using 1 tablespoon of dried nettles and 4 cups of water. However, let the infusion steep for at least 4 hours. Strain and drink to help ease the pain.

Headaches

Peppermint Oil

Peppermint essential oil or absolute can be used to help ease the pain of headaches. Make peppermint essential oil or peppermint absolute and add several drops to a tablespoon of olive oil to dilute. Rub directly on the temples to help remedy regular headaches.

Cayenne Poultice

This mini-poultice may seem strange at first, but once it gets rid of your headache once, you will swear by it forever. The poultice is made from cayenne pepper and water and is much more watery that a standard poultice. Mix ¼ teaspoon of ground cayenne pepper with 4 ounces of warm water. Swirl a cotton swab around in the mixture, making sure it is coated well. Rub gently just on the inside of the nasal passages until you can feel the heat from the pepper. You may feel a little burn, but once that subsides, so should your headache.

Feverfew Infusion

Feverfew can be beneficial in treating migraine headaches because it helps constrict the blood vessels and ease the pressure commonly associated with this kind of headache. Make a standard infusion using 1 ounce of dried feverfew flowers and 2 cups of boiling water. Steep for 10 minutes before straining. Drink half a cup twice a day

Ginger Root Infusion

Ginger Root can also be beneficial at fighting headaches. Make a standard infusion with 3 slices of fresh ginger root that are each about the size of a quarter and 2 cups of boiling water. Steep for 30 minutes, remove the solids, and drink.

Herbs that Help with Aches and Pains

Bay Laurel

Bay Laurel can be used to treat arthritic aches and pains, lower back pain, earaches, and sore muscles and sprains.

Camphor

Camphor oil helps to numb and cool the peripheral nerve endings when applied to the skin before warming the painful area by stimulating circulation in cold, stiff muscles and limbs.

Castor Oil

Castor Oil can be used externally for muscle and arthritis pain, bruising, and nerve damage.

Cayenne

Cayenne Pepper contains capsicum which can be beneficial in decreasing chronic pain including pain caused by arthritis and chronic nerve pain.

Clove Oil

Clove oil can be beneficial in treating dental pain. Add a few drops to a common ball and dab on the spot to help relieve toothache.

Devil's Claw

Devil's Claw can provide slow but effective relief to pain in the joints caused by all kinds of arthritis. It can also alleviate muscle pain.

Eucalyptus

Eucalyptus is generally used for congestion, but it can also be beneficial for relieving the pain associated with sore muscles and arthritis.

Feverfew

Feverfew has been an effective headache remedy for thousands of years. It can also be beneficial when used for the pain and inflammation of arthritis as well as to treat other types of aches and pains.

White Willow Bark

The origin of modern day aspirin, white willow bark is effective at treating pain and inflammation.

Yucca Root

Yucca has been shown to help with treating both osteoarthritis and rheumatoid arthritis.

Soothing Your Stomach

Stomach aches aren't fun for anyone, and these herbal remedies can help ease even the toughest tummy aches.

Chamomile Infusion

Chamomile helps alleviate stomach discomfort by easing inflammation and relaxing the muscles of the stomach. Make a standard infusion using 2 teaspoons of dried chamomile and 1 cup of boiling water. Steep for 20 minutes, strain, and then sip slowly.

Peppermint Infusion

An infusion made with fresh peppermint leaves can also help to soothe a sore stomach. It helps to relax cramping stomach muscles and can also help with gas and bloating. While you can also make this infusion with dried peppermint leaves, using fresh ones also allows you to munch on the steeped leaves which can provide additional benefit. Use a handful of fresh leaves or 2 teaspoons of dried leaves and 1 cup of boiling water. Steep for 10 minutes and sip.

Ginger Root Decoction

Ginger Root can also be beneficial for treating stomach aches and for relieving nausea. Make a standard decoction with 2 inches of fresh ginger root that has been peeled and finely chopped and 2 cups of water. Bring the water to a boil, add the chopped ginger root, and allow the water to boil for 3-5 minutes. Reduce the heat and simmer for 2-4 more minutes.

Remove from heat, strain out solids, and add a teaspoon of honey before drinking.

Herbs that Help with Stomach Problems

Caraway Seed

Caraway seed is effective at preventing gas and bloating. It can also help with colds and congestion and helps ease coughing by relaxing muscles.

Cardamom

Cardamom is similar to ginger and can also be beneficial in treating nausea including morning sickness.

Cinnamon

Cinnamon can be beneficial in treating digestive problems and upset stomachs.

Hops

When hops are fresh, they can be used to create bitters that help with digestion. When aged, hops can be used as sedatives.

Lemongrass

Lemongrass can be used to help treat nausea.

Other Top Herbs and Their Uses

Now that you have a basic understanding of the different ways herbal remedies are made and some examples of how they are used to treat common ailments, you can begin exploring how to use other herbal remedies to tend and mend your family's ailments and injuries. To help you in this exploration, here are the top herbs used to treat ailments in a variety of categories, so you have an idea of what you can use where as you begin creating your own remedies.

Aloe Vera Gel

The juice from the leaves of the aloe vera plant has important medicinal properties that can be used to burns and other ailments. It is often added to lotions, creams, and ointments because of its healing properties and is one of the most respected medicinal plants.

Boneset

Boneset, which comes from the medicine of the Native American tribes, can be beneficial in treating colds and fevers. It was the most popular treatment for these problems before aspirin.

Calendula

Calendula oil is your go-to remedy for minor first aid like cuts, scrapes, and bruises.

Lavender

Lavender has so many uses that it is like the jack of all trades of herbal medicine. It can be used to improve mood and sleep, alleviate pain, heal skin conditions like burns, and kill germs.

Witch Hazel

Witch Hazel can help with almost any problem on the skin. It's used in remedies to treat abrasions, burns, bites, and general skin inflammation.

Conclusion

I hope you found my *"Natural Cures"* guide helpful, and that it provided you with the foundation you need to start making your own herbal remedies at home.

When you can create many of the basic remedies your family needs to treat common ailments and injuries, you can save money, increase your self-sufficiency, and have the peace of mind of knowing what you are putting in your bodies.

You now have the know-how to start making your own herbal remedies from scratch using things you can easily grow in your own garden. You know:

- Why herbal medicine is a good fit for your family
- The benefits of herbal remedies
- How to make your own remedies
- The basic types of herbal remedies
- Herbal remedies for treating the common cold
- Herbal remedies for treating aches and pains
- Herbal remedies for treating stomach problems

You're now ready to start safely and inexpensively making your own herbal remedies at home.

Happy Homesteading!

Gaia

Check out some of Gaia's other books!!

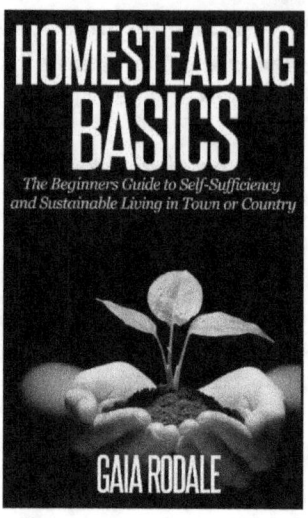

http://www.amazon.com/dp/B00JPVFVHC

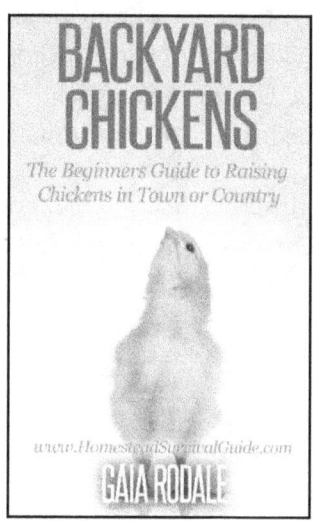

http://www.amazon.com/dp/B00KGLRRP4

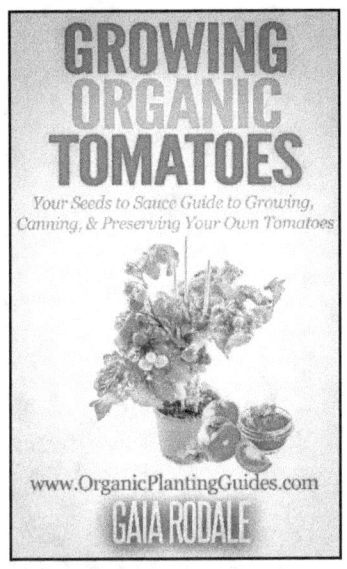

http://www.amazon.com/dp/B00K1FR7Y6

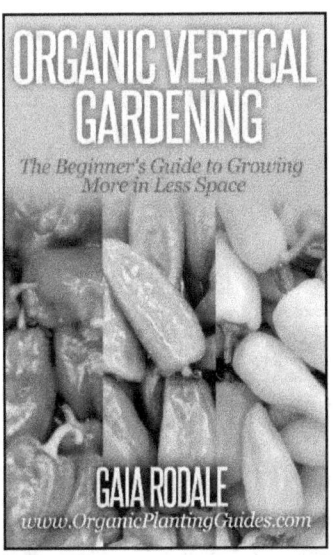

http://www.amazon.com/dp/B00KE8QM28

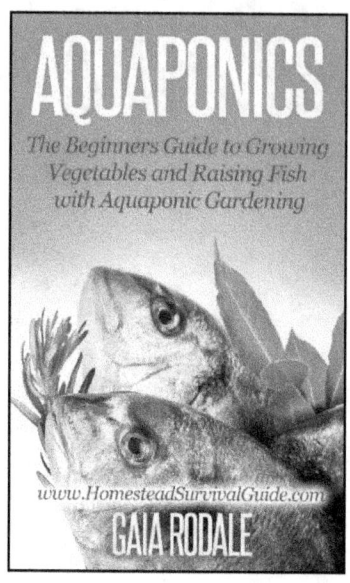

http://www.amazon.com/dp/B00KNFAWKU

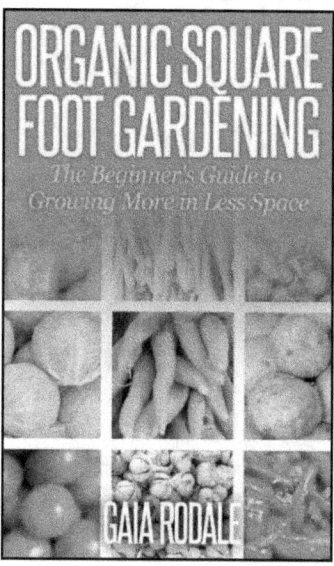

http://www.amazon.com/dp/B00JSA2JVG

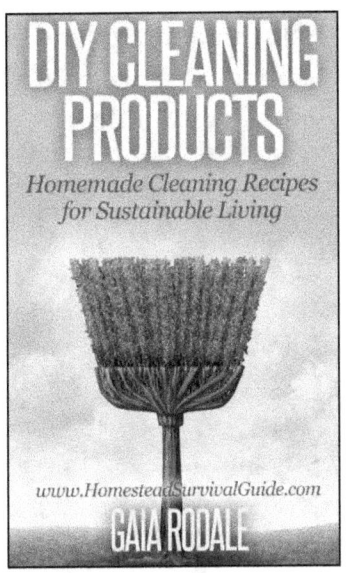

http://www.amazon.com/dp/B00L6EK8WY

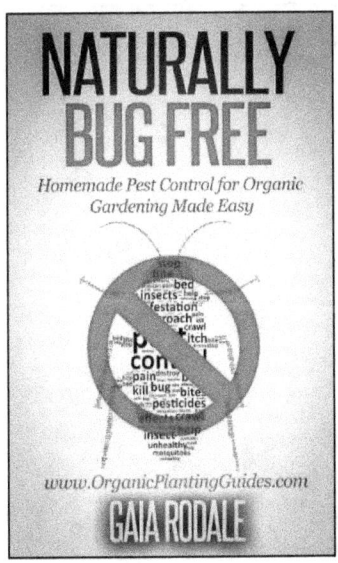

http://www.amazon.com/dp/B00L1WBQW2

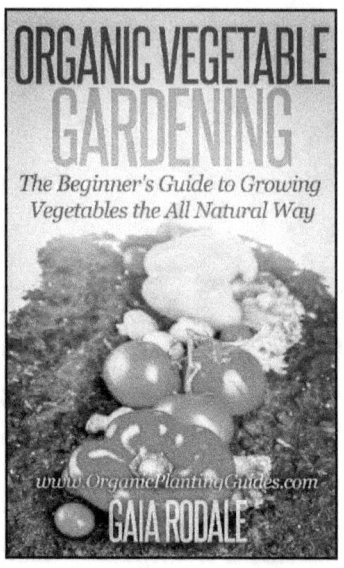

http://www.amazon.com/dp/B00KFXB7ZY

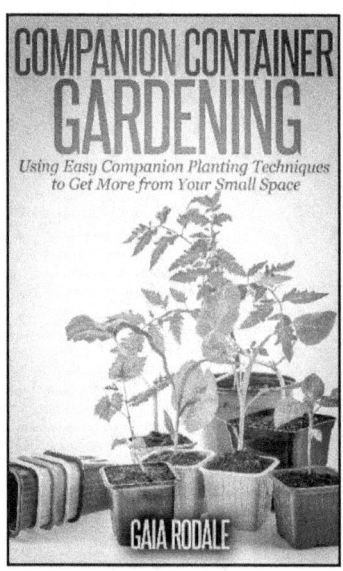

http://www.amazon.com/dp/B00J7ZUZOA

www.ingramcontent.com/pod-product-compliance
Lightning Source LLC
Chambersburg PA
CBHW070505290526
45790CB00003B/1099